1.877.JA

What Ar... Jay Robb's Fruit Flush?

Dear Jay,

I was shocked to see that I had lost 10 pounds *[on your FRUIT FLUSH™ plan]! I took your suggestion—and for 72 hours followed the FRUIT FLUSH™ and did not engage in any cardio or weightlifting exercises. During that period of time, I also experienced a mental and physical cleansing. This program provided me the jump-start I needed to take off the 10 pounds I packed on the past few months due to extensive traveling and a lot of fast food.*

—M.M., Birmingham, AL

I have been struggling for over a year to lose the weight I put on after having my baby. Jay Robb's FRUIT FLUSH™ 3-Day Detox program was the miracle I needed to gain the control I lost in my life—through increased energy almost overnight, toxic cleansing, and an organized easy way to transition back to a healthy lifestyle of optimum diet and nutrition. ***I lost 5 pounds*** *and overnight gained the confidence I needed to break my carb addiction. I am telling all my friends about this plan, Jay. I used to feel defeated;* ***now I feel empowered.***

—J.W., Cardiff by the Sea, CA

I completed the FRUIT FLUSH™ last week and ***lost 6 pounds in three days.*** *I felt so good after the diet that I didn't want to go back to eating junk food and drinking beer after work. My energy level has increased, and I am not feeling as tired as I was. I want to live a long and healthy life...this is a great place to start! Thank you, Jay! I wouldn't have been able to make these changes without your help.*

—R.S., Phoenix, AZ

The FRUIT FLUSH™ is part of my eating regimen now; I have followed it 4 times in two months, and the results have been amazing. Initially, ***I lost 9 pounds****—and every time thereafter,* ***I have lost 2-3 pounds from the cleansing.*** *This plan has been an eye-opener for me—as every time I cleanse and detoxify, my body shows signs that it is performing better. (This is especially important to me as I am 43 years old, a newlywed, and stepmother to two active boys.) I am sleeping better and am less fatigued on my busiest days when I am consuming the powder and eating a lot of healthy fruits. But the most significant impact on me is that I am developing new healthy habits that bless my family. Where I used to consider food shopping a hassle, I now enjoy finding great places to select fresh fish, fruit, and vegetables for my family. My attitude about caring for myself and my family has definitely improved!*

—H.G., Whittier, CA

As a 24-year old former modern dancer, I have to be very concerned with what I eat, how I feel, and how I look. My challenge is not losing weight—it is finding a plan that I can stay on that will allow me to attain optimum nutrition and performance. It has not been easy for me to find a program that offers a delicious menu and is easy to prepare and follow. That's why I enjoy Jay's FRUIT FLUSH™ program. It provides everything you need to cleanse, feel satisfied, detoxify, and lose weight at the same time! In just three days, ***I dropped 4 pounds*** *and feel like a new woman. I feel healthier, am thinking more clearly, and feel energized. I will never eat the way I did again. You would be amazed what a couple of days of fruit will do for you.*

—A.Y., Boynton Beach, FL

***I lost 6 pounds in three days**, and I was almost never hungry! Now I feel lighter than ever and am motivated to stick with eating a healthy diet. On the day after I finished the diet, I felt satisfied, didn't crave sweets, and ate healthy.*

—K.W., Pittsburgh, PA

*I completed the FRUIT FLUSH™ yesterday and **lost 5 pounds in just three days!** I feel terrific, my energy level has increased, and now I want to make a commitment to keep myself on track with The Fat Burning Diet. Your programs really work. I'm going to tell all of my friends. Thank you, Jay! I am appreciative that you were able to help me when others weren't.*

—S.R., Encinitas, CA

*Thank you, Jay, for creating healthy products and programs that my entire family can enjoy and follow. I just did your FRUIT FLUSH™ because I wanted to clean out my system—and actually **lost 8 pounds in the process!** I have been reading alarming statistics about cancer and am very interested in keeping my colon clean. I've always believed in taking preventive measures when it comes to my health. In fact, I started drinking your brand of whey protein shakes about a year ago when my friends raved about it. We have been buying tubs of your incredible tasting whey protein ever since. I am amazed at how smooth, full-bodied, and creamy your protein powder tastes—in just water and ice! (Most protein powders that contain stevia have a terrible aftertaste!) It's a great option for me "between meals" because it keeps my body feeling energized and stabilized.*

I am now reading your Fat Burning Diet book that has been recommended to me by a friend. Thanks for your great guidance and support, Jay. I'm a fan of yours for life!

—K.T., Oceanside, CA

I am a cosmetologist and single mother. I had been experiencing a lot of headaches due to stress. I heard about your FRUIT FLUSH™ and how it could help cleanse my body and help me feel better—so I gave it a try. I actually really enjoyed following the program. After the 3rd day, ***my headaches were completely gone****, I had more energy than before the detox program, and* ***I actually lost 4 pounds.*** *I feel like I can handle my life better now. Thanks, Jay.*

—D.P., Los Angeles, CA

I'm a personal trainer in Long Island, New York. I'm a subscriber of your newsletter, which I love, and I totally promote your products. I printed out your FRUIT FLUSH™ recently and gave it to a few of my clients. ***They loved it and lost weight easily****. We were all impressed with the diet and weight loss results. I will continue to recommend it to others. Keep up the great work, Jay!*

—L.A., New York, NY

The first time I did the FRUIT FLUSH™, I did it to slim down before a vacation. I lost 5 pounds. It was great. While in Mexico, I gorged on margaritas, pina coladas, lobster drenched in butter, and chips and guacamole. When I returned home, I got on the scale, only to find I gained back the 5 pounds, plus an additional 4! I started the FRUIT FLUSH™ immediately, on a Monday. By Tuesday, I was relieved to see that ***I lost 4 pounds the first day.*** *By the end of the 3rd day,* ***I lost 5 more—for a total of 9 pounds!*** *Jay, your FRUIT FLUSH™ will be a regular part of my routine to keep my eating habits clean!*

—T.R., Temecula, CA

Jay Robb
Certified Clinical Nutritionist

FRUIT FLUSH ™

3-Day Detox

Loving Health Publications
in conjunction with

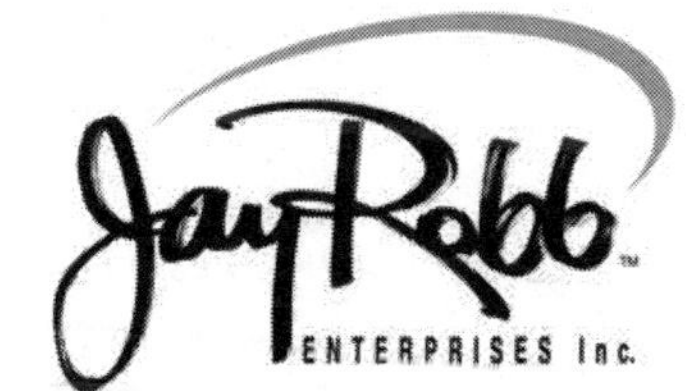

5670 El Camino Real, Suite C
Carlsbad, CA 92008

www.JayRobb.com / 1.877.JAY.ROBB

FRUIT FLUSH™ 3-Day Detox

Robb, Jay
FRUIT FLUSH™
3-Day Detox
Jay Robb

ISBN 0-9620608-8-7
1. Reducing diets. 2. Nutrition. 3. Diet—popular works.

Manufactured in the United States of America

Loving Health Publications
in conjuction with

Jay Robb Enterprises Inc.
5670 El Camino Real, Suite C
Carlsbad, CA 92008

Cover design by Jay Robb
Jay Robb's photo by Greg Aiken

Dedication

I dedicate this book to every person who wishes to take the first step towards getting in the best shape of their life—and to every person who has slipped into bad habits but desires to get back on track *fast.*

And a Very Special "Thank You"

—to my wife **Rosemary** and my son **Angelo** for your loving support at home. I love you both dearly and thank God every day that you are in my life!

—to our Public Relations Director, **Nancy Ferguson**, for going above and beyond the call of duty to help bring the FRUIT FLUSH™ to millions of individuals around the world.

—to our Editor / National Accounts Executive, **Heather Gervasi,** for doing double duty to help me complete this book and for always going the extra mile to support God's vision for this company.

—to the **entire staff at Jay Robb Enterprises Inc.** Many thanks to each member of the Jay-Team for offering your never-ending support to keep the office and warehouse running smoothly and efficiently. It is the combination of all of your god-given talents and time that has built, shaped, and made this company a huge success.

—to the **thousands of health food stores, gyms, nutrition and fitness centers, doctors' offices, and clinics across the nation** that carry our books and products. Your support is allowing us to reach and teach every man, woman, and child on this planet who desires to discover the health benefits of our nutriiton products and diet programs.

"Procrastination puts things off to a future time that doesn't exist. The only time to do anything is now."

—The Author

The author does not claim to be a doctor or healer of any sort. This book is intended for educational purposes only and should not be used as a guide for diagnosis and treatment of any disease. If you have any health problems, it is advisable to seek the advice of a health care professional of your choice.

Table of Contents

CHAPTERS: **PAGE**

> "Don't talk unless you can improve the silence."
> —Lawrence C. Coughlin

Introduction

"Purge your body of toxins, revitalize the mind, lose weight, and stay in tune with the Infinite."

Cleansing with natural foods has been a part of my life since the '70s when I gave up sugar, sweets, artificial sweeteners, chemical preservatives, refined foods, alcohol, and junk food. Up to that point in my life, my daily diet was dominated by white bread, burritos, and beer. The more junk I ate, the worse I felt. One day, I became sick and tired of feeling sick and tired and gave up my junk food cold turkey. The year was 1975, a pivotal point in my life. Utterly disgusted by the way I looked and felt, I gave up the sugar bowl, bread, and beer to embark on a lifetime mission of eating natural foods, lifting weights, and living a natural lifestyle. It was one of the best decisions of my life.

From 1975 to 1990, I experimented with a wide variety of diets. I also experimented with a wide variety of cleansing methods. During my experiments, I developed The Fat Burning Diet, which was first published nationally in 1991. At that time, I developed a unique cleansing program, which included the consumption of fresh fruits (eaten at regular intervals for one full day), and another program, which included the consumption of lean protein (also eaten at regular intervals for one full day). These two programs were the precursor to the FRUIT FLUSH™ program, which I personally use and advocate and will reveal for the first time in this book.

Cleansing is a regular part of my lifestyle. Cleansing with natural foods, especially fresh fruit, is a safe, fun, and easy way to keep your body fat levels low and your energy levels high. I have performed countless fruit flushes over the past 30 years. I perform them at various times throughout the year to tune up my body and flush away accumulated toxins in the cells, excess fat, and toxic waste matter that has stagnated in my colon.

I developed the FRUIT FLUSH™ 3-Day Detox program so that detoxifying the body can be as pleasant and easy as possible. Focusing on eating cleansing foods for just three days at a time is far more appealing than contemplating a cleanse that would last a week or longer. There are certain cases where a long-term cleanse would be called for (supervised by a health care professional), but, in most cases, the three-day FRUIT FLUSH™ is sufficient to purge the body of toxins, revitalize the mind, and stay in tune with the Infinite.

My FRUIT FLUSH™ is Ideal for Use if You Are:

- Wanting to drop three to nine pounds quickly and easily
- Getting ready to begin a new exercise program
- Getting ready to start a new diet
- Kicking off a new year
- Getting ready for a wedding
- Feeling toxic and bloated
- Experiencing constipation and gas
- Developing bags under your eyes
- Experiencing messy or foul-smelling bowel movements
- Ready for a change in lifestyle
- Getting ready for a dream vacation
- Addicted to carbohydrate
- Craving sugar and sweets
- Retaining water and fluids
- Partying too much
- Tired and depressed

God bless you,

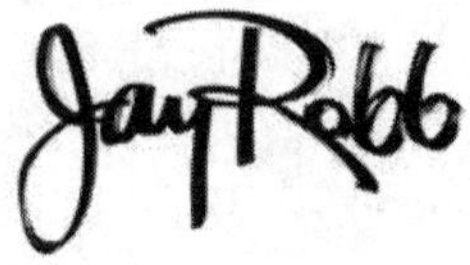

About Jay Robb

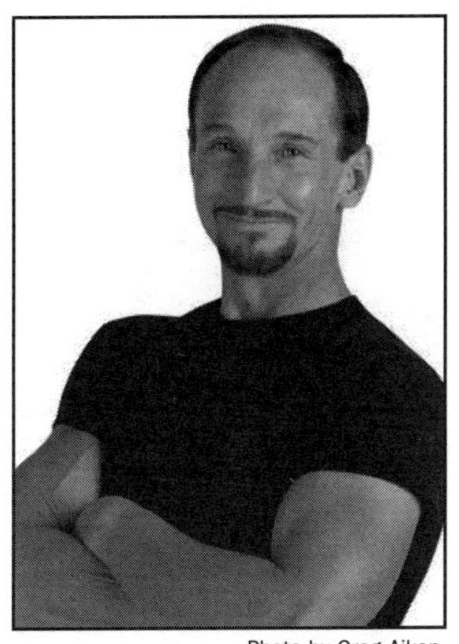

Photo by Greg Aiken

Jay Robb is a certified clinical nutritionist with over 25 years' experience as a professional in his field. He is the CEO of Jay Robb Enterprises Inc.—a multi-million dollar corporation (founded in 1988) that is famous for its high-quality, outrageously delicious protein powder formulas. Jay Robb products and books are sold in thousands of health food stores and gyms across the nation.

Jay is the author of the top-selling book *The Fat Burning Diet*, a feature columnist for *Natural Bodybuilding* magazine and *Best Body for Women*, and is a contributing writer for *Men's Exercise*, *Exercise for Men Only*, and various other national health and fitness publications.

The Jay Robb Corporation also produces the Jay Robb *Health-eNewsletter,* which is featured on the company website: www.JayRobb.com.

Jay Robb is dedicated to daily meditation and prayer, is happily married, has one son, and lives in La Costa, California—on San Diego's beautiful North County coastline.

"To experience reality, be still.
There is no other way."
—The Author

Chapter 1

Tune Up Before It's Too Late!

As a health and fitness professional, I have discovered over the past 25 years that the human body is a perfect design. The human body is a living machine that must be treated properly, which includes providing it with proper fuel and regular maintenance. In reality, your body is just like a car. If you put the proper fuel in a car, it performs at its best. If you try to cut costs and add water, dirt, cheap gas, kerosene, or the wrong fuel to your car's gas tank, its performance will drop or the car may even fail to start or run properly. Your car is also set up with a nice exhaust system. Your car ignites gasoline to power the engine then quickly removes the toxic residue from the cylinders by way of the exhaust system. Your car ignites the fuel and then pushes the exhaust down a long pipe and straight out the tailpipe. If anything goes wrong in the process, trouble will soon follow.

Imagine your car is not tuned up properly so the gasoline does not ignite fully and only part of the gasoline is burned. This creates a problem because now you have unburned gas in the cylinders—which is wasteful and contributes to air pollution. Now, imagine that you have a leak in your exhaust system and fumes are escaping into the car's interior. This problem can lower the car's performance and make you sick in the process. Now, imagine your car's tailpipe is plugged up and the exhaust can't escape. Within seconds your car's engine will die because it cannot operate unless the pollutants from the ignited gasoline are quickly removed.

FRUIT FLUSH™ 3-Day Detox

Your car's power system is like the power system in your body. If you give your body the wrong fuel, your performance drops and you risk toxic buildup from the residue of unburned or improperly burned fuel. If your tailpipe (colon) is plugged up, the residue of the foods you are eating and the toxic byproducts of normal metabolism cannot be evacuated; hence you can become ill from toxic overload.

As a clinical nutritionist, I could try to impress you with medical terms, big words, and fancy jargon. But you might miss the real message in the process of me "wowing" you with my knowledge of human anatomy. Instead of using complex medical terminology, I have written this text for the layman, using analogies that are easy to understand and grasp. Eating a healthy diet is not rocket science; neither is detoxifying the body of pollutants. In reality, the laws of Nature do all the work. All you need to do is give your body the opportunity to cleanse itself. That's it.

To cleanse and detoxify your body does not require that you ingest some special drug, consume four cups of organic oat bran daily, or drink a tea from a rare herb that only grows on the backs of female tortoises on the Galapagos Islands. Nor should you have to torture yourself by purging and cleansing for months and months to make your innards squeaky clean. Cleansing can be quite easy and fun if you understand the basic principles of the process.

Cleansing is actually a daily process that keeps your body slim and operating at optimum efficiency. The key to successful cleansing is to allow your body to detoxify itself regularly by eating properly and to also perform periodic fruit flushes to super-clean your system. The FRUIT FLUSH™ is here to help you do all that and more so you can have a trim body that is free from toxic overload, free from disease, and overflowing with vital energy. My friend, it is time to cleanse!

Chapter 2
Are You Toxic?

"The time to take action is *right now*.
There is no other time."
—The Author

YOU MAY BE TOXIC IF:

- You consume diet drinks, soft drinks, coffee, tea, or alcoholic beverages.

- You eat white bread, white buns, sugar, doughnuts, cakes, pies, ice cream, candy, sugared gum, white rice, and refined foods.

- You are constipated and/or have gas, bloating, or indigestion.

- You lack energy, feel lethargic, lack stamina, and often procrastinate.

- You are depressed, anxiety ridden, sad, or have lost your zest for life.

- You need to wear glasses or contacts.

- Your bowel movements are messy and require lots of toilet paper to clean up after.

- Your tongue is coated, your eyes are bloodshot, or you have bags under your eyes.

• Your blood sugar levels are high or you have developed type 2 diabetes, hypoglycemia, or chronic fatigue syndrome (CFS).

• Your body temperature is regularly below 98.6 degrees Fahrenheit during the day.

• You find it difficult to stick with an exercise program, job, or any task at hand.

• You are moody and your mind sometimes races out of control.

• You have trouble sleeping and/or wake up feeling tired.

• Your sexual performance or sex drive is lagging.

• You are addicted to carbohydrate-rich foods—such as sweets, bread, pizza, cookies, and junk food.

• You feel weak and shaky if you go without eating for over four hours between meals.

• You must consume snacks, sweets, sodas, or coffee to give you a lift between meals.

• You crave certain foods and must have them each day to feel right.

• You are overweight or underweight.

• Your mind is foggy and/or your memory is poor.

• You have trouble focusing or have attention deficit disorder (ADD) or attention deficit hyperactive disorder (ADHD).

• Your lower abdomen is bulging, yet little fat can be grabbed around your midsection.

- You do countless sit-ups or crunches—yet you still have a fat, bloated stomach.

- You consume recreational or prescription drugs on a regular basis.

- Your occupation or environment places you in contact with toxic substances.

- You smoke cigarettes, cigars, a pipe, or chew tobacco.

- You drink less than three quarts of water a day.

- You do not fast or cleanse your system regularly.

The bottom line is: Nearly every person on this earth is potentially toxic. Americans—experiencing a dramatic decline in overall health, preoccupation with drugs, and the chronic consumption of junk food—just may be the most toxic group of people on the planet! If you are overweight, lack energy, and suspect your body is overloaded with toxins, then it is time to cleanse your system now!

The ultimate FRUIT FLUSH™ 3-Day Detox program was created so that you can periodically pro-actively help purge unwanted debris from your mind and body. Your body and mind are interconnected. If your body is toxic, so are your thoughts. It is a natural result. If your body is swimming in a cesspool of waste, then your thoughts will reflect this foulness. People who are toxic seem to share certain characteristics. It is not uncommon for a toxic individual to be self-centered and experiencing some mental and/or physical pain. It is also not uncommon for them to swear frequently and speak negatively. Their glass is usually half empty instead of half full.

"It has been my observation that most people get ahead during the time that others waste."
—Henry Ford

Chapter 3
Fruit Power!

"Never purchase beauty products in a hardware store."
—Miss Piggy

Fresh fruit is Nature's perfect cleansing food. Fruit grows abundantly in most warm regions of our planet. Man is basically a tropical animal. He has no fur to protect him from temperatures below 50 degrees Fahrenheit; hence he is designed to ideally live in tropical and subtropical parts of the world. Because man is a cunning species, he has learned to create artificial tropical regions all over the planet. In other words, he has never really left the tropics. We, humans, just keep creating miniature tropical environments wherever we choose to live.

In the United States, people living in the northern states are subjected to extreme temperatures plunging below zero degrees Fahrenheit during the winter months. The animals that are adapted to living in this climate have thick layers of fat on their bodies and/or thick fur coats. We don't have enough body fat to keep warm in cold climates, nor do we sport a thick coat of fur to protect us from old man winter. But we do have the creative wisdom to build homes that are heated to 70 degrees Fahrenheit, to build cars with heaters that boost the temperature inside to 70 degrees Fahrenheit, and to build sky rise office buildings that are heated to 70 degrees Fahrenheit. We have even created clothing (including those made with animal furs) to keep the air next to our skin approximately 70 degrees Fahrenheit.

In the coldest climate, we can still wake up in a tropically warm environment and rinse our naked skin under a makeshift tropical waterfall—that we refer to as a *shower*. Our skin adapts to the sun by becoming darker to protect us from overexposure, which is how we have evolved and adapted to the tropical sun. If humans had slowly migrated north over a period of thousands or millions of years, the human body would have adapted to cold climates by developing a thick layer of subcutaneous fat and a thick fur coat. We just never have had to adapt to a harsh climate because we are still living in the tropics, no matter where we choose to live. Instead of the body physically adapting, we have altered our immediate surroundings so that we are always living in a tropical climate.

Fruit grows in abundance in the tropics and is a food that man is well adapted to consuming. Many fruits have seasons, especially in the subtropics. Therefore, when specific fruits come into season, man gorges on them; then Nature takes them away. Over time, other fruits come into season; and their seasons end. In the tropics, some fruits produce year-round (like bananas and papayas), while other fruits (like mangos) have definite seasons.

Fruit is high in water content, high in fiber, and high in natural slow-releasing sugars. The nutrients in fruit help dissolve toxins, and the water and fiber in fruit helps flush out toxins by way of urine and bowel. The sugar in fruit is of a unique nature. It actually breaks down slowly into glucose because the fructose fraction must first be converted in the liver. A meal of fresh fruit can require up to an hour and a half for the sugars to fully convert to glucose and fill the bloodstream. Fructose, found in fruit, is also the preferred sugar for replenishing liver glycogen.

The human body contains approximately 350-400 grams of carbohydrate stored as glycogen. Approximately 100 of those grams are stored in the liver with the remainder residing in the muscles. Glycogen is the body's reserve source for carbohydrate. When consumed in adequate amounts, fresh fruit could easily keep glycogen levels filled while also supplying one's daily carbohydrate needs.

Have our bodies ever *really* adapted to anything but a tropical diet that includes fresh fruit, coconuts, fish, vegetables, nuts, and seeds? Your body has no way of knowing that it is not living in the tropics, no matter where you currently live. As tropical animals, fruit is very well suited for our bodies, and it pleases our palate. Eating a substantial quantity of fresh fruit periodically can do wonders for an overfed, undernourished body. The periodic consumption of fresh fruit can also naturally supply the body with vitamin C, flush the colon, cleanse the tissues, cleanse the lymph system, rinse away excess sodium, and pep up one's spirits.

> "For life to be a dream come true, it is critical to know who is dreaming."
> —The Author

Chapter 4

The FRUIT FLUSH™ 3-Day Detox

Four Ways to Utilize the FRUIT FLUSH™ 3-Day Detox:

NOTE: On the days you are not performing the FRUIT FLUSH™, consume healthy foods according to the principles outlined in Jay Robb's book, *The Fat Burning Diet.*

1. **FRUIT FLUSH™ FOR FAT LOSS:**
Perform the three-day FRUIT FLUSH™ once a week for up to 12 consecutive weeks. This will have you cleansing and revitalizing your body three out of seven days each week for up to 12 straight weeks. If you are cleansing to lose weight on this program, you should lose up to 9 pounds the first week and 2 pounds each week thereafter, until you reach your goal weight.

2. **FRUIT FLUSH™ FOR LIFE:**
Perform the FRUIT FLUSH™ once or twice a month throughout your lifetime—if you so desire.

3. **FRUIT FLUSH™ TUNE-UP:**
If you have slipped off your diet and/or have been eating the wrong foods (i.e., during the holidays or at special events), then the FRUIT FLUSH™ is a great way to quickly cleanse your system and get you back on target.

4. **FRUIT FLUSH™ FOR A FRESH START:**
Prior to beginning an exercise program or starting a new diet, you may want to cleanse your body first with the FRUIT FLUSH™. It can get you off to a great start!

How to Perform the FRUIT FLUSH™:

Day 1: PRE-FLUSH

Mix 1 ¼ cup of whey protein or egg white protein powder (your flavor of choice) with 1 quart (32 ounces) pure water. Shake, blend, or stir, and store in a sealed container in a cool place. The protein powder you choose must NOT BE sweetened with added carbohydrate or contain artificial sweeteners. This means it MUST NOT CONTAIN: aspartame, fructose, sucrose, evaporated cane juice, sucralose, maltodextrin, sugar, corn syrup, corn sweeteners, barley malt, molasses, agave, or brown sugar. The protein powder you choose should also contain approximately 24 grams of protein per one-ounce serving. If you choose an egg white protein, you may wish to add the herb stevia to naturally enhance the perceived sweetness without increasing carbohydrate content. Before pouring each glass of protein as outlined below, lightly shake or stir the container to re-mix the protein drink.

SHOPPING TIPS: Choose a high-quality protein powder that tastes good. Avoid the bargain brands that may save you a buck or two but can taste like chalk and are often filled with aspartame, sucralose, fructose, sugars, acesulfame-K, acesulfame potassium, and artificial flavors and colors. The body is a temple of the spirit. It deserves only the best. *I also suggest purchasing organically grown foods whenever possible.*

8AM 6-oz glass of protein mix
10AM 6-oz glass of protein mix
NOON 6-oz glass of protein mix
2PM 6-oz glass of protein mix
4PM 6-oz glass of protein mix
6PM 3-6 cups raw vegetable salad *and* 3-6 oz of lean chicken, fish, turkey, or beef <u>or</u> scramble 4-8 egg whites in 1 tsp olive oil. Top the salad with 1-2 tbs olive <u>or</u> flax seed oil (or ½ avocado) and the juice of ½ lemon or lime.

NOTE: Drink an 8- to 12-ounce glass of water one hour after you consume each protein drink or meal. (If this doesn't quench your thirst, you may consume more water.)

Days 2 and 3: FRUIT FLUSH™

8AM 1 serving fresh fruit
10AM 1 serving fresh fruit
NOON 1 serving fresh fruit
2AM 1 serving fresh fruit
4PM 1 serving fresh fruit
6PM 3-6 cups raw vegetable salad. Top the salad with 1-2 tbs olive or flax seed oil (or ½ avocado) and the juice of ½ lemon or lime. Consume 1 protein drink mixed, as follows:

- 12 oz pure water
- 5 tbs high-quality whey or egg white protein powder
- Stir and drink slowly

NOTE: Drink an 8- to 12-ounce glass of water one hour after you consume each fruit meal. (If this doesn't quench your thirst, you may consume more water.)

Days 2 and 3: FRUIT FLUSH™ MEAL IDEAS

8AM 2 cups cantaloupe, honeydew, or watermelon
10AM 2 medium oranges
NOON 2 medium apples
2PM 1 cup fresh pineapple
4PM 1 medium banana
6PM 3-6 cups raw vegetable salad. Top the salad with 1-2 tbs olive or flax seed oil (or ½ avocado) and the juice of ½ lemon or lime. Consume 1 protein drink mixed, as follows:

- 12 oz pure water
- 5 tbs high-quality whey or egg white protein powder
- Stir and drink slowly

AN IMPORTANT NOTE ABOUT FRUIT: Some nutritionists believe in only eating low-carb or low-glycemic fruits due to the belief that sweet fruits, such as bananas and grapes, can overload the system with sugar. Because you are only eating one serving of fruit every two hours and it is a fact that fructose enters the bloodstream at a relatively slow rate, on the FRUIT FLUSH™, you may confidently choose whatever whole, fresh, raw, natural fruit you choose without fear of overloading your system. Juice is NOT ALLOWED on the FRUIT FLUSH™, nor is dried fruit, both of which are too concentrated for use with this program. Avocados, which are rich in fat, are only allowed in the evening with your salad.

Fresh Fruit Serving Sizes for Reference:

THE FOLLOWING LIST CONSTITUTES APPROXIMATELY 1 SERVING (100 CALORIES):

Apples	2 medium
Apricots	6 medium
Banana	1 medium
Blackberries	1.5 cups
Blueberries	1.5 cups
Cantaloupe	2 cups cubed
Cherries	1 cup
Grapefruits	2 large
Grapes	1 cup (or 15-18 grapes)
Honeydew	2 cups cubed
Kiwifruits	2 medium
Mango	1 large or 2 small
Nectarines	2 small
Oranges	2 medium
Peaches	3 medium
Pears	1 medium
Pineapple	1 cup
Plums	3 medium

Raspberries	1.5 cups
Strawberries	2 cups
Tomatoes	4 medium
Watermelon	2 cups (cubed or balled)

During the entire three days of the FRUIT FLUSH™, you should become slightly hungry every 2 hours, at which time you will eat. This eating pattern fuels your body and keeps you from ever being overly hungry. On Day 1, the series of protein drinks will stoke your metabolism, lower your glycogen levels, and force your body to burn fat as part of its energy needs. On Days 2 and 3, fruit will power your body while cleansing and purifying the cells and organs. Plus, the protein drinks and fresh fruit are high in water content, which, in turn, will help keep your system hydrated.

FRUIT FLUSH™ Shopping List:
(Purchase organic foods when available.)

___ 16 oz whey protein or egg white protein powder

___ Fresh fruit of choice

___ Raw salad vegetables (variety is important)

___ 1 avocado (if used as a salad topping)

___ Olive oil or flax seed oil (for salad dressing)

___ 2 lemons or limes

___ 1-2 gallons pure water

___ 3-6 oz chicken, fish, turkey, or lean beef

___ 4-8 egg whites (if you prefer, in place of lean chicken, fish, turkey, or beef)

> "Many of us don't realize that what we eat greatly determines how we look, which may explain why I once looked like a jelly-filled doughnut."
>
> —The Author

Chapter 5

Post-Flush Principles to Stay Regular

"Nearly any disease can be due to a toxic colon."
—Robert Gray

After each FRUIT FLUSH™, it is important to eat a wholesome diet according to The Fat Burning Diet principles. I have also created a fantastic new **"Colon Rejuvenating Drink"** that can be taken once before meals 3 times daily to improve regularity and colon health. This cocktail is a high-fiber lactobacteria food designed to feed the friendly bacteria in your colon at high speed while sweeping away toxic debris, cholesterol, and waste matter.

My Colon Rejuvenating Drink is very effective because it combines two powerful ingredients—sweet dairy whey and psyllium seed husks—that synergistically recondition your colon. The sweet dairy whey feeds the lactobacteria in your colon, and the psyllium seed husks act as a soothing fiber to help cleanse the colon walls.

Consuming Jay Robb's Colon Rejuvenating Drink 3 Times Daily Before Meals Can Help Produce:

- Regularity
- Nearly odorless bowel movements
- Easy-to-pass stools
- Improved digestion
- A healthy immune system
- Improved colon health

Recipe for Jay Robb's Colon Rejuvenating Drink:

In a 10-ounce glass of water, add the following ingredients (or mix ingredients into your protein drink):

- 2 tbs psyllium seed husks
- 2 tbs sweet dairy whey
- If desired, you may add a pinch of stevia to enhance flavor

Stir and drink within 30 seconds. If you mix these ingredients in a protein drink, it will create a creamy smooth drink that is rich in taste and fiber.

NOTE: Sweet dairy whey is rich in lactose, which can rapidly feed the lactobacteria in your colon. If you are lactose intolerant, this product may cause you to have gas, feel bloated, or get intestinal cramps. If you have any doubt, test the sweet dairy whey by consuming only 1 teaspoon per drink, and work up slowly over a period of 30 days or more to 2 tablespoons per drink. If you discover that sweet dairy whey does not work for you (a small percentage of the population may be severely lactose intolerant), then substitute the sweet dairy whey with an inulin powder, which is a unique fiber source that can also feed lactobacteria in the colon (inquire at your local health food store for its availability). Inulin, in my experience, is not nearly as effective as sweet dairy whey for building a high lactobacteria population but is a viable alternative for those few who are severely lactose intolerant.

Questions and Answers

"God *is* the answer. What is the question?"
—The Author

FRUIT SUGAR RUSH?
Q. Fruit is high in sugar. Will eating that much fruit cause blood sugar problems during the FRUIT FLUSH™?

A. *Fruit is a perfect food for human consumption. Fructose, the main sugar in fresh fruit, requires up to 90 minutes to fully reach the bloodstream. This process is relatively slow because fructose must be shuttled to the liver to be converted to glucose, thus naturally helping you avoid a sugar rush. In fact, fruit is such an ideal food and enters the bloodstream so gradually that it does not cause a rapid rise in glucose or give you that sleepy feeling 30 minutes after a meal—as can a plate of pasta or any refined starchy carbohydrate. Despite popular belief, whole fresh fruit will not give you a sugar rush when eaten in moderation.*

PROTEIN POWDER PREFERENCES?
Q. Can I use the whey protein powder I have in my kitchen cabinets? It contains acesulfame-K and fructose, but the rest of the ingredients look okay.

A. *No! Do not use a protein powder that contains acesulfame-K or fructose. Use only a protein powder that is free of sweeteners, including artificial sweeteners.*

Here is a list of ingredients to avoid in a protein powder. The protein powder you choose should provide, in a single serving, 24 grams of protein per ounce (28.35 grams).

INGREDIENTS TO AVOID:
- Casein
- Calcium caseinate
- Sodium caseinate
- Fructose
- Aspartame
- Acesulfame-K
- Acesulfame potassium
- Sucralose
- Sugar
- Sucrose
- Evaporated cane juice
- Artificial flavors and/or colors

CONSTIPATION RELIEF?
Q. I am currently constipated. Will the FRUIT FLUSH™ help me attain regularity?

A. *Being regular will require more than the FRUIT FLUSH™ 3-Day Detox, but you can expect to expel some of the stagnant matter from your colon during the cleanse. Fruit is an excellent food for moving sluggish bowels into motion. For tips on getting your colon in shape, please refer to Chapter 5 in this book and to Chapter 13 in my latest edition of The Fat Burning Diet.*

WILL I DEVELOP GAS?
Q. I am frequently plagued with gas and bloating. Will your FRUIT FLUSH™ program give me gas or make me feel uncomfortable?

A. *I have carefully designed the FRUIT FLUSH™ to digest in a manner that should not cause gas and/or bloating. Of course, to rid your body of old stagnant waste matter, you may experience some mild gas as the fruit stirs up the toxic debris and* *pushes it through your body.*

IS THE FRUIT FLUSH™ PROGRAM OKAY FOR DIABETICS?
Q. I am a type 2 diabetic. Can I perform your FRUIT FLUSH™ program?

A. *You should have no problems following this program for three days, but please check with your doctor first. It is important to check your glucose levels throughout the day during the entire program and utilize insulin, if needed, on the fruit days. Day 1 is a low-carb day, so your insulin needs may only be minimal. Again, check with your doctor before starting the program.*

WHAT ABOUT HYPOGLYCEMIA?
Q. I have hypoglycemia. Won't eating all that fruit upset my blood sugar levels?

A. *Not at all. In fact, most of those suffering with hypoglycemia actually have developed food allergies and are also operating with weakened adrenal glands—both of which can lead to unstable blood sugar levels. I developed severe hypoglycemia in the '70s yet experience no symptoms today or at any time when I am fruit cleansing. I have the most blood sugar problems when I eat wheat, whole grains that contain gluten, and refined carbohydrates.*

IS THE FRUIT FLUSH™ GLUTEN-FREE?
Q. I am gluten intolerant. Does your diet contain any foods that contain gluten?

A. *I, too, am gluten intolerant. Gluten is a protein found in most whole grains. Millions of Americans may be gluten intolerant. The symptoms are chronic gas, bloating, constipation, and diarrhea, following the consumption of whole grains that contain gluten. Wheat is the most common and richest source of gluten in the American diet. Wheat is everywhere and seems to be in everything we eat. The FRUIT FLUSH™ program is wheat- and gluten-free so you may utilize it without reservation.*

WHAT ABOUT SOY PROTEIN?

Q. I notice that you only recommend whey or egg white protein powders be used to make the protein drinks. Can I use a soy protein powder?

A. *Yes. You can use a soy protein powder as long as you know you are not allergic to soy and the soy protein is not sweetened. Soy is not digested properly by certain individuals, and many others are actually allergic to soy products—so I always caution its use. If you try using a whey or egg white protein and they don't work well for you, you may then want to try a high-quality soy protein. I don't suggest soy protein for men because it may lower sperm activity, according to recent research.*

WHAT IF I AM UNDERWEIGHT?

Q. I am underweight. Will your FRUIT FLUSH™ program make me lose more weight? I can't afford to get any thinner.

A. *If your weight is already down to a minimum, then you will probably not lose much weight, if any, during the program. After the FRUIT FLUSH™, you may notice that you will gain weight easier (healthy muscular weight) due to an internally cleaner body and a more powerful digestive system.*

LOW THYROID?

Q. My thyroid activity is low. Will your FRUIT FLUSH™ further decrease my thyroid function?

A. *Hypothyroidism can be caused by many factors—including low-protein intake, iodine deficiency, stress (a huge factor), a diet that is too low in carbohydrate, and a diet that is too low in calories. My FRUIT FLUSH™ program is designed to cleanse the body, using foods as the cleansing agents. Because this program lasts only three days, you probably will not experience any change in your thyroid activity, but each individual varies. I suggest you consult with your physician if you have any concerns about your condition.*

INTERCHANGING OF THE MEALS?

Q. Can I consume the dinner suggestions at lunchtime and consume the protein drinks or fruit in the evening?

A. *No. The program is designed to cleanse the body at maximum efficiency by eating the foods in the exact order listed each day. Changing the order of the foods consumed could hinder the cleansing power of the program.*

WHAT ABOUT SUPPLEMENTS?

Q. Can I take my nutritional supplements during the FRUIT FLUSH™ 3-Day Detox program?

A. *No. Except for the use of a protein powder, you will not be taking additional nutritional supplements. You may resume your normal supplementation regimen immediately following the three-day cleanse.*

DAIRY PRODUCT SENSITIVITIES?

Q. I am allergic to "all dairy" products. Can I still perform your FRUIT FLUSH™ program?

A. *Yes! Whey protein is a dairy product; however, most individuals who are sensitive to dairy products are actually allergic to casein, thc protein in milk, and not to whey protein. You can test whey protein, and if you are sensitive to it, then use egg white protein instead. The rest of the diet is 100% dairy-free.*

WHAT ABOUT MEDICATIONS PRESCRIBED BY MY DOCTOR?

Q. Should I continue to take my medications during the FRUIT FLUSH™ 3-Day Detox program?

A. *Yes. It is important that you continue taking all of your prescribed medications, unless otherwise directed by your physician. If you have any doubts or questions, please consult with your doctor.*

HOW YOUNG?

Q. My daughter is 14 years old and is about 10 pounds overweight. Can she perform your FRUIT FLUSH™ program?

A. *Yes! My program may be utilized the entire three days by anyone who is 12 years or older and in good health.*

CLEANSING NONSTOP?

Q. If I am doing great on your FRUIT FLUSH™ program, can I repeat the program immediately following the completion of the three days?

A. *No! The FRUIT FLUSH™ is designed to be used a maximum of three days per week. If you were to continue on without a break, you may run the risk of experiencing some unpleasant cleansing reactions. The beauty of the program is how comfortable, pleasant, and easy it is to cleanse your system periodically. Just be patient, and utilize the program only once per week. On the days you are not following the program—to get maximum results—I suggest you follow the dietary principles outlined in my book, The Fat Burning Diet.*

BAD BREATH?

Q. My wife and I experience bad breath from time to time. What causes this, and will your FRUIT FLUSH™ help us eliminate this problem?

A. *Bad breath, medically termed "halitosis," can be caused by one or more of the following things: a faulty diet, poor digestion, poor gum health, poor dental hygeine, food allergies, and a low lactobacteria count in the colon. In my opinion, the most offensive form of halitosis is caused by poor digestion of certain foods (usually dairy products) and a low lactobacteria count in the colon. In my own experience with bad breath, I discovered I do not properly digest casein, which is the protein found in milk, cheese, and many other dairy products (but not in whey protein). When casein fails to break down properly, it can ferment in the gut; hence the fermentation is noticed on the* *breath as a bad odor. This problem can be accelerated when milk and cheese are consumed with fruit or any form of concentrated sugar. As a clinical nutritionist and in my 25 years as a health and fitness professional, I have encountered many, many clients who do not digest milk products (casein) properly, and the result is bad breath. By simply removing milk and cheese from their diet, the bad breath usually disappeared. Yogurt, which is a predigested milk product, does not cause this problem nor does whey protein (which is usually free from casein) or sweet dairy whey. Because the FRUIT FLUSH™ is virtually "casein free," anyone with casein-induced halitosis should see it clear up after just one day on the program.*

SAFE FOR PREGNANCY?

Q. I am pregnant. Is it okay to perform your FRUIT FLUSH™ during my pregnancy?

A. *No. During pregnancy you are eating for two, and performing a cleanse that induces weight loss is not advised. I do recommend those who are wishing to become pregnant to perform the FRUIT FLUSH™ as a means of cleansing the body in preparation for conception.*

WHAT IF I AM BREASTFEEDING?

Q. My son was born six weeks ago, and I am still breastfeeding him. Can I perform your FRUIT FLUSH™?

A. *Yes, but please check with your doctor first. Breastfeeding, like pregnancy, means you are eating for two. In general, you should do very well on the FRUIT FLUSH™ during breastfeeding because only natural foods are on the FRUIT FLUSH™ menu. If you become tired by Day 3 of the FRUIT FLUSH™, then rest more. It is also best not to repeat the FRUIT FLUSH™ more than two times each month until you stop breastfeeding.*

CAN I DRINK MORE WATER?
Q. Can I drink more water than you suggest in the FRUIT FLUSH™?

A. *You may drink as much pure water as you desire on the program. DO NOT add anything to this water. It must be pure mountain spring water, distilled water, reverse osmosis, or filtered water only. Sparkling water must also be avoided.*

WHAT ABOUT HEADACHES?
Q. During the first day of the FRUIT FLUSH™, I developed a mild headache that lasted throughout the afternoon and into the early evening. Does this mean I was detoxifying my body?

A. *Mild headaches are common the first day of cleansing for those who regularly consume coffee, tea, or caffeine-laced soft drinks. Detoxification headaches are also common for those who may have hidden food allergies to everyday foods—such as bread, wheat, cereals, grains, and milk—none of which are on the FRUIT FLUSH™ menu.*

NO-CALORIE SODAS?
Q. Can I drink no-calorie sodas and soft drinks during the FRUIT FLUSH™?

A. No! Calorie-free soft drinks are usually laced with aspartame, acesulfame-K, sucralose, artificial flavors, artificial colors, and other potentially toxic ingredients. I don't recommend these types of drinks. If a low-calorie sugar-free soft drink is desired during times when you are NOT performing the FRUIT FLUSH™, I suggest purchasing sparkling water and adding a twist of lemon or lime and a pinch of the herb stevia to naturally duplicate the taste of a regular or diet soda. Try it, you'll like it!

CAN I USE A PROTEIN POWDER WITH VARIOUS FLAVORS?
Q. Jay, I love the taste and quality of your whey protein powder. Most of the protein powders I have tried in the past contain ingredients that I don't wish to put into my body, plus they often taste gritty or chalky. Your protein is the best I have ever found. Can I use any and all of your many flavors of whey protein on the FRUIT FLUSH™?

A. *Thank you for your kind words about our whey protein. Yes, you may choose any of our six outstanding flavors (vanilla, chocolate, strawberry, pina colada, tropical dreamsicle, and watermelon). Our unflavored whey may also be used on the program.*

CAN I DRINK COFFEE ON THE FRUIT FLUSH™?
Q. I like to have one or two cups of coffee in the morning to wake me up. Can I still have my coffee while following your FRUIT FLUSH™ program?

A. *No! Coffee contains the drug caffeine and should not be used on the FRUIT FLUSH™. Caffeine is an addictive drug that millions of Americans are addicted to. The FRUIT FLUSH™ is designed to help individuals break their addiction to caffeine and other drugs. After three days on my program, individuals often feel empowered to eliminate bad habits because they feel so fantastic after cleansing their system.*

CAN I DRINK TEA OR HERBAL TEAS ON THE FRUIT FLUSH™?
Q. I like to drink a cup of herbal or regular tea several times a day. Can I use either of these on the FRUIT FLUSH™?

A. No! Regular tea (unless decaffeinated) contains caffeine which is not allowed on the program (for more on this, see previous Q and A). Herb teas (which I believe to be medicinal and acceptable for occasional use when not following the FRUIT FLUSH™) are not allowed on the program because some herb teas can be aggressive cleansers of the body. The FRUIT FLUSH™ packs enough cleansing power on its own without the use of herb teas. If one begins cleansing too fast, he or she can experience toxic overload. Also, some herb teas can cause allergic reactions and/or can be stimulating, further making them unsuitable for use on the FRUIT FLUSH™.

SHOULD MY HUSBAND EAT MORE BECAUSE HE IS BIGGER?
Q. Should my husband increase portion sizes on the FRUIT FLUSH™ because he weighs well over 200 pounds?

A. *No! I have carefully designed the FRUIT FLUSH™ to work for everyone, large or small. The regular feedings of specific foods allow the body to cleanse itself of toxins and excess sodium while maintaining stable blood sugar levels.*

CAN I TAKE EXTRA FIBER ON THE FRUIT FLUSH™?
Q. I add oat bran each day to my morning cereal to supply my body with extra fiber. Can I use added fiber while following the FRUIT FLUSH™?

A. *No! While I am an advocate of eating a high-fiber diet and ingesting additional fiber daily to ensure colon health, I do not allow additional fiber to be used on the FRUIT FLUSH™. The FRUIT FLUSH™ contains ample fiber that is naturally occurring. I am also not a fan of using wheat bran, oat bran, or any whole bran from grains because they can be irritating to the colon and small intestine. I recommend psyllium seed husks combined with sweet dairy whey as the preferred combination of a natural fiber and lactobacteria food for use AFTER the FRUIT FLUSH™ (for more on fiber and regularity, see Chapter 5).*

PROTEIN BAR SUBSTITUTION?
Q. Can I eat protein bars instead of the whey or egg white protein drinks?

A. *No! Many of the protein bars on the market contain "junk" ingredients and should be avoided during the FRUIT FLUSH™. After the FRUIT FLUSH™, you may once again resume eating protein bars. But take great care in selecting bars that DO NOT* *contain acesulfame-K, sucrose, sucralose, fructose, high-fructose corn syrup, corn sweeteners, aspartame, evaporated cane juice, casein, sodium caseinate, artificial flavors, and artificial colors.*

WHAT ABOUT EXERCISING?

Q. Can I exercise during the three days I am following the FRUIT FLUSH™ program?

***A.** Yes, but make it light and simple. FRUIT FLUSH™ is a detoxification program. During the three days that you follow the plan, it is best to rest more which will allow your body to cleanse itself. If you feel weak or tired while following the FRUIT FLUSH™, then heed the signs and REST. Many individuals are exhausted because they are toxic and overstimulated from the regular use of coffee, tea, and stimulating drinks. If you feel strong and want to exercise while following the FRUIT FLUSH™, then please do so but don't overdo it. Walking is a great exercise to perform during the 3-Day Detox. You may also enjoy swimming, weightlifting, bicycling, and other forms of exercise, but please keep it light and lively. If your body indicates that it is tired, then relax, put your feet up, read a book, or get more sleep.*

CAN I SALT MY FOODS?

Q. I love salt and would like to use it during my three days on the FRUIT FLUSH™. Can I freely salt my foods because salt contains no calories?

***A.** No! While salt is an essential mineral that is important to good health, most individuals ingest way too much sodium each day in the form of table salt and/or sea salt. If taken in excessive amounts daily, salt can cause your body to excrete potassium and upset your delicate electrolyte balance. The FRUIT FLUSH™ is designed to help you excrete excess sodium while ingesting foods that are high in potassium to help rebalance your system and rid yourself of excess water that you may be retaining. (Sodium must be suspending in water, so excess* *sodium can cause you to look and feel bloated because you are holding onto excess water.)*

WHAT ABOUT USING VINEGAR?

Q. In place of the lemon or lime juice over the salad as part of the salad dressing, may I use apple cider vinegar instead? Many health books advocate the use of apple cider vinegar for its many health benefits.

A. *No! For some individuals, apple cider vinegar can be a wholesome addition to a salad, while others may have an allergic reaction to vinegar. Apple cider vinegar is a fermented product that contains yeast. Millions of individuals around the world may be allergic to or sensitive to yeast and can have a negative reaction when they ingest yeast containing foods. Because the FRUIT FLUSH™ is designed to allow the body to cleanse itself, apple cider vinegar is not allowed due to its fermented properties and yeast content. After completing the FRUIT FLUSH™, you may use apple cider vinegar on your salad and see if you react to it. If no reaction occurs after two back-to-back meals containing apple cider vinegar, you can assume it is safe to use periodically, as desired. If you DO react to apple cider vinegar, it may be best to avoid it for several months, then retest it again.*

For more information, visit JayRobb.com, or call toll-free 1.877.JAY.ROBB.

> "Try turning on a light before complaining about being in the dark."
> —The Author

Be a FRUIT FLUSH™ Superstar!

Send us your FRUIT FLUSH™ success story, and you may be selected to be featured on Jay Robb's Website.

Once you have experienced the weight loss and cleansing power of the FRUIT FLUSH™, take a few minutes to send us your success story. If your story and photo are selected, you could be seen by millions of people around the world. We want to congratulate you on your success and are offering you an opportunity to inspire others to make positive changes in their life.

It's Easy to Submit Your Story:

1. Write your success story (100 words or more), and explain, in detail, why you performed the FRUIT FLUSH™, how much weight you lost, and how this experience has changed your life.

2. Include a photo of yourself after completing the FRUIT FLUSH™. You may dress any way you choose for this photo, but it is suggested that you wear clothing or a swimsuit that makes you look your absolute best.

3. Email your success story and photo (as a JPEG) to FruitFlush@jayrobb.com.

God bless you and good luck!

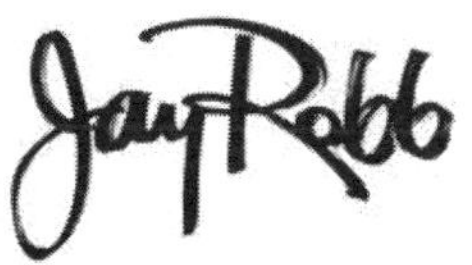

Other Popular Works by Jay Robb

Certified Clinical Nutritionist

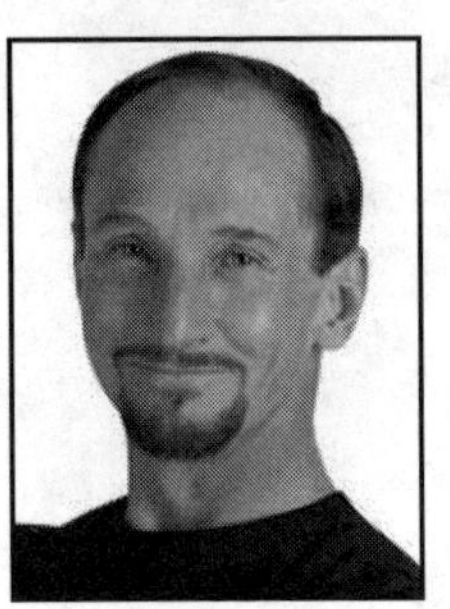

The Fat Burning Diet
(Discover how Jay Robb kissed diabetes, hypoglycemia, depression, fatigue, and excess body fat good-bye!)

The Fat Burning Diet Cook Book
(Over 150 mouthwatering fat burning recipes!)

Secrets to Staying Slim (CD)
(Lose excess fat like never before!)

Jay Robb's FREE Health-eNewsletter
(Stay on the cutting edge of health and fat loss!)

Fit for Christ
(How to realize that God is everything!)

For more information:

1.877.JAY.ROBB / JayRobb.com

Bibliography

Bengmark S. 2003. Use of Some Pre-, Pro- and Synbiotics in Critically Ill Patients. *Best Pract Res Clin Gastroenterol* 17(5):1-15.

Brand-Miller J, Hayne S, et al. August 2003. Low-Glycemic Index Diets in the Management of Diabetes: A Meta-Analysis of Randomized Controlled Trials. *Diabetes Care* 26(8):2261-2267.

Crook, M.D., WG. 1991. *The Yeast Connection.* Professional Books 2-3.

Edwards AJ, Vinyard BT, et al. 2003. Consumption of Watermelon Juice Increases Plasma Concentrations of Lycopene and B-Carotene in Humans. *J Nutr.* 133:1043-1050.

Erasmus, U. 1990. *Fats that Heal—Fats that Kill.* Alive Books.

Farnsworth E, Luscombe ND, Noakes M, et al. 2003. Effect of a High-Protein, Energy-Restricted Diet on Body Composition, Glycemic Control, and Lipid Concentrations in Overweight and Obese Hyperinsulinemic Men and Women. *Am J Clin Nutr.* 78:31-39.

Fiocchi A, Martelli A, et al. July 2003. Primary Dietary Prevention of Food Allergy. *An Allergy Asthma Immunol.* 91:3-13.

Forman, Ph.D., Robert. 1977. *How to Control Your Allergies.* Larchmont Books 186.

Gray, R. 1983. *The Colon Health Handbook.* Rockridge Publishing Co. 17.

Jensen, D.C., B. 1981. *Tissue Cleansing through Bowel Management.* Jensen 74-75.

Johnston, I. and J. 1990. *Flaxseed (Linseed) Oil and the Power of Omega-3.* Keats Publishing 23.

Layman DK, Boileau RA, et al. 2003. A Reduced Ratio of Dietary Carbohydrate to Protein Improves Body Composition and Blood Lipid Profiles During Weight Loss in Adult Women. *J Nutr.* 133:411-417.

Linskens RK, Huijsdens XW, et al. 2001. The Bacterial Flora in Inflammatory Bowel Disease: Current Insights in Pathogenesis and the Influence of Antibiotics and Probiotics. *Scand J Gastroenterol.* 36(Suppl 234):29-40.

McNamara D. May 15, 2003. Regular Breakfast Eaters at Lower Risk for Obesity. *Family Practice News* 10.

McNamara D. July 2003. Vitamin C Derivative Cleared More Acne than Clindamycin 1%. *Skin and Allergy News* 36.

Maynard M, Gunnell D, et al. 2003. Fruit, Vegetables, and Antioxidants in Childhood and Risk of Adult Cancer: The Boyd Orr Cohort. *J Epidemiol Community Health* 57:218-225.

Nelsen DA. December 15, 2002. Gluten-Sensitive Enteropathy (Celiac Disease): More Common than You Think. *Am Fam Physician* 66(12):2259-2266, 2269-2270.

Pereira MA, Liu S. 2003. Types of Carbohydrates and Risk of Cardiovascular Disease. *J Women's Health* 12(2):115-122.

Plaskett LG. September 2003. On the Essentiality of Dietary Carbohydrate. *J Nutr Environ Med.* 13(3):161-168.

Santillo B.S., M.H., H. 1987. *Food Enzymes, The Missing Link to Radiant Health.* Hohm Press 2.

Seccareccia F, Alberti-Fidanza A, et al. Vegetable Intake and Long-Term Survival Among Middle-Aged Men in Italy. *Ann. Epidemiol* 13(6):424-430.

Suga A, Hirano T, Kageyama H, Osaka T, Namba Y, Tsuji M, Miura M, Adachi M, Inoue S. April 2000. Effects of Fructose and Glucose on Plasma Leptin, Insulin, and Insulin Resistance in Lean and VMH-Lesioned Obese Rats. *Am J Physiol Endocrinol Metab* 278(4):E677-E683.

Waring WS, Goudsmit J, Marwick J, et al. November 2003. Acute Caffeine Intake Influences Central More than Peripheral Blood Pressure in Young Adults. *Am J Hypertens* 16(11 part 1):919-924.

Webster, D. 1995. *Achieve Maximum Health: Colon Flora-The Missing Link in Immunity, Health & Longevity.* Hygeia Publishing.

Wurtman, J.J., Ph.D. 1986. *Managing Your Mind and Mood through Food.* Rawson Associates 21-23.

Wurtman RJ, Wurtman JJ, et al. 2003. Effects of Normal Meals Rich in Carbohydrates or Proteins on Plasma Tryptophan and Tyrosine Ratios. *Am J Clin Nutr.* 77:128-132.

Yang EJ, Chung HK, et al. 2002. Carbohydrate Intake Is Associated with Diet Quality and Risk Factors for Cardiovascular Disease in U.S. Adults: NHANES III. *J Am Coll Nutr.* 22(1):71-79.